Autism

The Ultimate Handbook To
Parenting And Teaching An
Autistic Child That Will Improve
Their Lives Forever.

by Suzanne Jensen

Published in United States by:

Suzanne Jensen

© Copyright 2015 – Suzanne Jensen

ISBN-13: 978-1515325116
ISBN-10: 1515325113

Table of Contents

Introduction

The main reason behind writing this short book on children with Autism Spectrum Disorder (ASD) is not to educate people about autism, but to let all people know how to make life easier, simpler, and better for children affected with this tough disorder that makes learning and development a big challenge.

The primary objective is to educate the families and caregivers (at home and school), difficulties they face and how we can help them make their days, weeks, months and years smoother. And you can only do so if you know the difficulties that they face. Let us find out.

The three main areas of impairment are social skills, communication, and behavior. Let us find out why.

Social skills: These children sometimes face difficulties interacting with peers and friends, both at school and outside. They face issues picking up social cues and understanding situations. In social situation, this child may either withdraw or display unusual responses. When they do engage with someone socially, it is often found that they lack the imaginative qualities and some aspects of social engagement.

Communication skills: Children affected with ASD have difficulties their feelings and needs verbally and/or non-verbally. They also have difficulties with non-verbal behavior like eye contact, use of pictures, gestures, facial expressions, etc. They often use repetitive and (apparently) unusual behavior.

Behavior: They often show obsessions or preoccupations with specific themes and objects. Often, they like order and may do things repetitively. They may behave unusually at times. For instance, they might suddenly start rocking, or start flapping their arms. They face difficulties whenever the time comes for a change in their schedules and may need some time to adjust to the change.

Again, some or most of the children affected have difficulties understanding sarcasm and other social behavior. The above list is by no means a complete list of difficulties faced by children affected by this disorder.

As far as cognitive development is concerned, some of these children may display almost normal capabilities, and some of them may lag way behind. It is important to understand that the learning capabilities and sensibilities of all children vary and each one of them is different. In fact, no two of children affected with ASD are same.

So, first let us learn a bit more about ASD and find out how to make life better for them as and when we interact with them.

Chapter 1:
What Is Autism?

In fact autism is not a single condition. One can say that there are different kinds of autism. That is why it is referred to as Autism Spectrum Disorder (ASD). ASD is a general term that includes conditions like Autistic disorder, Asperger disorder, and Pervasive Developmental Disorder-Not otherwise Specified (PDD-NOS), Childhood disintegrative disorder, and Rett's disorder (in females).

Children diagnosed with ASD face difficulties in the following areas:

- Communication and language
- Socialization
- Restricted interests, and

- Repetitive behavior.

Within the above areas, many different symptoms are manifested by ASD patients. Therefore two different ASD patients usually have a different set of behaviors and abilities.

The range of ASD symptoms is a broad one. Some speak in single words or short sentences, while some have great verbal skills. Some children are less sociable and like to be alone, while some like to socialize, but face challenges in socializing.

These children have a wide range of interests and repetitive behavior. Some children have interest in unusual things like signboards, street signs, animals, plants, gardens, etc., while some have made it a hobby of collecting unusual objects like pencil sharpeners, erasers, etc.

In some cases, the interests of these children may not be appropriate for their age and in terms of the intensity as well. For instance, a child has a knack for detailed information on a particular topic and sometimes, they are known to have extreme interest in only one item (like an unhealthy interest on one particular toy above all others).

Another common observation is that they have repetitive behaviors/mannerisms. They may be simple behaviors like flapping of their hands or a more complex mannerism. The list may be endless.

It important thing is to remember and keep in mind that each child with ASD is unique and no two children would behave like each other. So, there is a need for personalized care for each ASD patient.

Roughly 1 out of every 85 children is born with ASD and boys are 5 times more likely to be affected than girls, going by the numbers.

Early Indicators of Autism

In the event that you think your kid may have Autism Spectrum Disorder, please read through the rundown of conceivable indications of ASD.

Your kid does not have to exhibit the greater part of the showed practices to be alluded for an appraisal.

Kindly note that these qualities might likewise be markers of different conditions. Conceivable early indications of ASD

(a) Impairment in Social collaboration

- Lack of fitting eye look
- Lack of warm, cheerful expressions
- Lack of offering interest or happiness
- Lack of reaction to name

(b) Impairment in Communication

- Lack of indicating signals
- Lack of coordination of non-verbal correspondence
- Unusual prosody
- Little variety in pitch
- Odd inflection
- Unpredictable mood
- Surprising voice quality

(c) Repetitive Behaviors as well as Restricted Interests

- Repetitive developments with items

- Repetitive movements or posing of body

In the event that your kid demonstrates two or a greater amount of these signs, please approach your pediatric human services supplier for a referral for an assessment. A screening apparatus called the M-CHAT (Modified Checklist for Autism in Toddlers) can likewise help you figure out whether an expert ought to assess your youngster. This straightforward autism screen takes just a couple of minutes. In the event that the answers recommend your tyke is at danger for a mental imbalance, please counsel with your kid's specialist. In like manner, in the event that you have some other worries about your youngster's advancement, don't hold up. Address your specialist now about screening your kids.

Individuals with a type of Autism, called mentally unbalanced savantism, have outstanding aptitudes in particular territories, for example, music, craftsmanship, and numbers. Individuals with this type of a mental imbalance have the capacity to perform these abilities without practice or lessons.

Warning Signs That Your Child May Have Autism?

Children create at their own particular pace, some more rapidly than others. Then again, you ought to consider an assessment for Autism if any of the accompanying apply:

- Your youngster does not coo or babble by 12 months of age

- Your little baby does not motion, for example, point or wave, by 12 months of age

- Your kid does not say single words by 16 months

- Your kid does not say two-word states on his or her own (as opposed to simply rehashing what another person says) by 24 months

- Your kid has lost any dialect or social abilities (at any age)

- Your kid does not build or keep up eye contact

- Your tyke does not make outward appearances or react to your outward appearances

Factors that are Responsible for Autism

There is no known single reason for a mental imbalance disorder or autism, yet it is for the most part acknowledged that it is brought about by anomalies in cerebrum structure or capacity. Cerebrum sweeps show contrasts fit as a fiddle and structure of the mind in youngsters with a mental imbalance contrasted with in neurotypical kids. Specialists don't have the foggiest idea about the precise reason for a mental imbalance yet are exploring various speculations, including the connections among heredity, hereditary qualities and medicinal issues.

In numerous families, there seems, by all accounts, to be an example of autism or related handicaps, further supporting the hypothesis that the issue has a hereditary premise. While nobody quality has been recognized as bringing on autism, specialists are hunting down sporadic fragments of hereditary code that youngsters with a mental imbalance may have acquired. It additionally creates the impression that a few kids are conceived with a weakness to a mental imbalance, however analysts have not yet distinguished a solitary trigger that causes autism. Different analysts are exploring the likelihood that under specific conditions, a bunch of precarious qualities may meddle with mind health, bringing about a mental imbalance. Still different analysts are researching issues amid pregnancy or conveyance and in addition ecological elements, for example, viral contamination, metabolic lopsided characteristics and presentation to chemicals.

Genetic Vulnerability: A mental imbalance has a tendency to happen more habitually than anticipated among people who have specific medicinal conditions, including delicate X disorder, tuberous sclerosis, innate rubella disorder and untreated phenylketonuria (PKU). Some unsafe substances ingested amid pregnancy additionally have been connected with an expanded danger of Autism.

Ecological Factors: Examination shows different variables other than the hereditary segment are adding to the ascent in expanding event of autism – for instance, ecological poisons like overwhelming metals, for example, mercury, which are more predominant than previously. Those with autism (or those at danger) may be vulnerable against such poisons, as their capacity to metabolize and detoxify these exposures may be compromised.

Some other theories on Autism:

- The invulnerable framework of body might improperly deliver antibodies that assault the brains of kids, creating a mental imbalance. This hypothesis is not generally considered as being legitimate.

- Anomalies in cerebrum structures cause extremely introverted conduct.

- Youngsters with a mental imbalance have irregular timing of the development of their brains. Right on time in adolescence, the brains of youngsters with autism become speedier and bigger than those of typical kids. Later, when ordinary youngsters' brains show signs of improvement composed, the brains of children with autism become all the more gradually.

Can Childhood Vaccines be Responsible for Autism?

There is no proof that any immunization can bring about Autism or any sort of behavioral issue. A suspected connection between the measles, mumps, rubella (MMR) immunization and Autism was proposed by a few folks of kids with a mental imbalance, yet all around reported boundless studies have marked down any affiliation. One premise for the dismissal of the hypothesis is that ordinarily, manifestations of a mental imbalance are initially noted by folks as their tyke starts to experience issues with postponements in talking after age one. The MMR antibody is first given to kids at 12 to 15 months of age; Autism cases with an evident onset inside a couple of weeks after the MMR inoculation might basically be an inconsequential chance event.

Hypothesis that an additive utilized as a part of immunizations, thimerosol, is in charge of an increment in a mental imbalance cases has additionally prompted studies that have demonstrated no proof of a connection.

The disorders within the autism spectrum

The disorders included in ASD are as follows:

Autistic disorder

Children affected by Autistic disorder face issues forming normal relationships and communicating with others. Their range of interests and activities are limited. Symptoms vary greatly between patients. Strangely, numbers of boys affected by Autistic disorder are five times that of girls.

Asperger disorder

Also called Asperger syndrome also affects more boys than girls. Asperger patients have normal intelligence and their language capabilities develop early. However, their social skills are impaired and cannot communicate effectively with others. Children with Asperger disorder are known to have poor coordination, repetitive speech, difficulties with reading comprehension, maths, written skills, obsession with some specified topic and lack of common sense.

PDD-NOS

Pervasive Developmental Disorder-Not otherwise Specified (or PDD-NOS) is called atypical autism. It is a neurological disorder that has some but not all attributes of Autistic Disorder. Children with PDD-NOS are known to have severe impairment in several spheres of development.

Childhood Disintegrative Disorder

This is a condition that occurs in 3-4 year olds. The child's intellectual, social and language skills are hit and deteriorate over several months. It is also called Heller's syndrome. Symptoms include loss of social skills, loss of bowel and bladder control, loss of motor skills, and delay or lack of spoken language skills, inability to start and sustain oral communication, etc.

Rett's disorder

This is seen in girls (mostly) between age of 6 and 18 months. It is characterized by wringing of the hands, slow head and brain growth, seizure, walking abnormalities, and mental retardation.

How Autism is diagnosed?

On the off chance that an autism side effects are display, the specialist will start an assessment by performing a complete therapeutic history and physical and neurological exam. Albeit there are no research facility tests for a mental imbalance, the specialist may utilize different tests -, for example, X-beams and blood tests - to figure out whether there is a physical, hereditary, or metabolic issue creating the manifestations.

On the off chance that no physical issue is found, the tyke may be alluded to an authority in youth advancement issue, for example, a youngster and pre-adult specialist or therapist, pediatric neurologist, formative behavioral pediatrician, or another health proficient who is extraordinarily prepared to diagnose and treat a mental imbalance. The specialist constructs his or her analysis with respect to the kid's level of improvement, and the specialist's perception of the youngster's discourse and conduct, including his or her play and capacity to associate with others. The specialist frequently looks for data from the kid's guardians, educators, and different grown-ups who are acquainted with the kid's indications.

The diagnosis process deliberately surveys social and relational abilities, confined and redundant intrigues and stereotyped examples of conduct.

The indicative appraisal incorporates:

- An exhaustive guardian meeting utilizing the Autism Diagnostic Interview
- Formal perception utilizing the Autism Diagnostic Observation Schedule
- Casual perception in common settings like the tyke's preschool or school where conceivable
- An input session delineating the evaluation results, including an open door for addressing and illumination
- Suggestions for administrations that will best serve the individual needs of the individual getting the determination
- Exhaustive composed report inside one month of the evaluation date
- For somebody who may have autism, a positive determination can help them and those near to them to comprehend the practices that were separating, befuddling and regularly disquieting.

Youthful youngsters who are diagnosed with autism have the capacity to get to the sorts of administrations that can essentially enhance their prospects for an important life. Youths and grown-ups, who may have masked or made up for their correspondence or different disabilities preceding the judgment, have the capacity to get to administrations that will bolster their capacity to communicate socially, enhance their business opportunities and their capacity to have important connections.

How to boost security inside and outside homes of ASD affected children

While every child is different, some children suffering from ASD have little or no sense of danger and can be impulsive. These children are prone to wandering away from your sight and may cause harm to themselves when unsupervised. Some steps that may be of help are:

- A fence around your backyard or pool.
- Attach alarms to the windows, door, gates close to stairs, guardrails of your child's bed and childproof latches on cabinets.
- Ensure small objects are beyond their reach and know how to give CPR (cardio pulmonary resuscitation) and first aid.
- Have audio monitors all over your home.
- Best to have someone watching your child if possible.

Children with ASD are known to be attracted to water sources like pools, ponds, etc., and drowning is the leading cause of accidental death of children suffering from ASD. Put together an information packet and give it to the police, neighbors, and other relevant people. This handout should include your child's picture, height, weight, distinguishing marks, address and all relevant phone numbers like yours, your wife's, etc. Make sure it also indicates how your child communicates.

If your child cannot communicate, consider having him wear an identification bracelet with his name, home phone number, etc. Chances of accident dip when hazardous objects at home are labelled with 'NO' or 'STOP' stickers.

Educating and handling a child with special needs

An Individualized Education Program (IEP) is a document that details the child's education. It is an educational program that should be tailored for individual students to provide maximum benefits. Since we are dealing with autistic children here and their needs vary individually, the word 'individual' is the key here.

The plan outlines the following:
- The special education plan for the child (goals

for the year)
- Services that are needed to assist the child meet these goals
- A method to evaluate progress made by the child

I am sure that most of my readers would be aware of that already.

Chapter 2:
Learning Needs Of Asd Affected Children

Children with ASD experience different thought processes and emotions. We need to make small adaptations to set them up for success. Let us find out a little bit about the difficulties faced by a child with ASD.

- They display poor organizational skills,
- Are not adequately rewarded by the normal social interactions around schoolwork,
- Expectations from them need to be spelled out very clearly,
- They cannot predict how long an activity would last,
- Are not sure when to start or end something (which in part makes them display repetitive behavior),

- Have trouble determining the order in which things need to be done,
- Have an impaired sense of anticipation and have trouble expecting things like we do,
- They are troubled by uncertainty and thus unable to concentrate on the task at hand.

Visual techniques are needed to individually strategize and enhance their learning process and for that reason, the role of the parents and caregivers become vital to their success.

Some strategies to help children with ASD complete assigned tasks are discussed below.

Workload

It is important that these children are given easily achievable workloads. They should also be made to choose. For instance, they can be made to choose the rewards for completing a task. There should also be a definite end to their work, and it should be clearly stated to them. Otherwise, they tend to repeat even the tasks they have done.

They should to follow a schedule as well. For example, give them worksheets stacked one above the other. This way, they know that they have to complete x number of worksheet to complete a task.

You may introduce the child to time bound tasks

with the help of an analogue clock, like, for instance, explaining to them that task a needs to be completed before the big hand gets to 4.

The tasks

The tasks assigned to a child should ideally be a healthy mix of tough, unfamiliar tasks along with some easy and familiar tasks the child likes. That helps take the stress off learning.

Present same tasks in different ways. Boredom and monotony is always an issue with children with ASD. Use the child's interests more imaginatively. For instance, paste an image of his favorite cartoon at the corner of a new worksheet. That lends a calming effect to a demanding situation.

Balance tasks keeping in mind the interest levels of the child. For example, keep a healthy mix of tasks with high, medium or low interest jobs throughout the day.

Include tasks that are relevant and functional as far as possible. They would resist tasks that have no clear meaning or relevance to them. And every task should have a clear starting point and a definite end point as well. The child needs to know the target or the reason he is doing something.

The ideal environment

Allocate specific areas for specific tasks. Use visual schedules that he clearly understands. Understanding sequence is the key to being a good learner. There are ways to achieve this and we would talk more about that later. Always make sure that the child is aware of what is expected of him.

Instructions, feedback and rewards

Verbal instructions can sometimes be open to misinterpretation. For instance never say draw a rectangle and not a square. The child might just end up hearing the square. Keep it simple. Just say 'draw a rectangle'. Always be crystal clear.

Demonstrate when teaching something rather simply explaining it. Use visuals whenever possible. Children with ASD respond better to visual cues.

Use a trial and error method to find out the reward that best motivates the child. Have a rewards list compiled. Various things may motivate various children. It is not like one size fits all. The rewards should be functional, concrete and should provide immediate gratification to the child. And most importantly, change rewards frequently.

Schedules

Schedules and procedures and sequences are a big challenge for these children. Their understanding of the concept of time is not the same as us. They have a more limited understanding. The same applies to predicting order, sequencing, and organizing things.

Another difficulty is that these children face is communication, specifically verbal instructions. Change creates stress in their minds and ASD affected children are more comfortable with the rigidity and sameness of their lives.

Most children with ASD are visual learners and respond better to visual cues rather than verbal commands. Visual methods of imparting instructions may include, but are not limited to computer generated graphics, written words, visual instruction via blackboards or white boards, photographs and comic strips, etc.

The schedules are the cornerstones of effective management of children with ASD. They are used to set limits, explain the concept of start and finish, and explain what change means. Schedules can be used to develop comprehension, and also used as opportunities to interact and communicate.

Transition strategies

By transition, I mean joining new school, starting interaction with a new teacher, joining a new class in school, and all other activities that begin with a change in ways of life for the children. Changes, irrespective of whether they are big or small, give rise to anxiety, confusion and other issues which have to be dealt with as and when they occur.

- Any type of change, like changes in teachers, classroom, playground, books, a new principal, etc. can cause anxiety in your child. Here are some tips to deal with them.

- Use a new set of visual timetables or visual cues to indicate any change.

- Schools should notify the parents before any major changes and if possible, discuss the lifestyle changes with the children's parents.

- Use photographs as far as possible, like a picture of your child's new school, teacher, playground, class, or co students.

- The child should be aware of the strategies to stay calm, like listening to music on a Walkman or mobile phone, or a favorite book, or a toy like a Rubik's cube. Or simply, when upset, the child can be taught to spend time in a quiet area.

- Similarly, allocate an area where the student will go to if lost at any point of time in school. Choose a convenient place you are sure to have some adults manning the area. Do the same for the neighborhood and inform local people, police, security guards etc.

- If your child has problems with organization, you can

have active strategies to aid him in that case, like putting materials for different classes in separate sub containers within his school bag.

- Allocate a specific area of the playground for your child to play if needed.
- Always ensure that a proper channel of communication exists between parents and teachers at school. Like a journal or a diary for instance where anything of note can be updated.

Chapter 3:
Strategies For Teaching Social Skills

The whole idea behind this chapter is to make parents and caregivers aware of the difficulties faced by the child with ASD as far as learning social skills are concerned. Socializing is normal and inborn for most of us, but unfortunately, it does not come naturally to those with ASD. The areas of difficulty for them are:

- Interaction with others
- The concept of a Code of conduct
- Friendship and kinship
- Eye contact with others, and
- Emotion.

It is an all pervasive difficulty that covers all aspects of their lives and they have to be taught social skills specifically. Their lack of social judgement can be displayed in many ways like shouting and interrupting a classroom session inappropriately, speaking to peers and teachers in the same tone without recognition to their status, inappropriate comments on somebody's appearance and actions, sticking to rules too rigidly, interpreting language literally, difficulty in initiating and continuing friendships, understanding that same behavior can be acceptable or unacceptable under different conditions, etc.

A good caregiver (I would like to include teachers and care providers at home under this category as well) should be aware of certain things like:

- What upsets a particular child,
- How to establish a working and pleasant relationship with the child based on routine. Consistency is the key here and a caregiver should always use similar, understandable and consistent ways to make the child aware whether he has done a good job or not,
- Carefully plan and use real life situations to explain concepts to the child,
- How to make a child adapt to one on one situation, small groups or classroom situations,
- Encourage the child to develop an ability to understand situations, accept change and ask for help

as and when needed and stay near the child when he is likely to be confused, and

- Involve other people like peers, school staff, parents etc. with the tasks assigned to them. This helps them learn social rules.

Remember, that each child affected by ASD is differently abled and teaching every autistic child is not the same. However the general ways guidelines remain the same and the caregiver needs to use the trial and error method to gauge individual capabilities. Some of the social skills that need to be ingrained to these children are:

- Greeting other people,
- Initiating and ending social interactions,
- Choosing activities,
- Sharing,
- Waiting,
- Taking turns,
- Playing games, etc.

Greeting other people

How to greet people they come across socially is one of the most important lessons a child with ASD has to be taught. While shaking hands is ideal for some situation, it is hardly so when meeting peers, teachers should be accorded more respect, while greeting family members properly is altogether different. At home and school, the caregiver should point out and reinforce these differences.

Situations keep happening when teaching these children how to greet properly. For instance, school staff walking briskly down the corridor may greet your child and he takes 10 to 20 seconds to respond. The caregivers must be patient enough to wait.

Initiating and ending social interactions

A social script can be useful in this case. A child should be able to categorize the people they meet into friends, acquaintances, etc. Social scripts break down situations into steps and clearly outline what is expected of the child in very clear terms like rules of behavior and good manners. We shall talk more about social scripts later.

That is why schools are important. Pupils should be taught how to enter and exit a play situation, how to receive and initiate an interaction with peers, what to say when you meet someone and how to say goodbye properly.

Choosing activities

Transitions between activities are anxious moments for ASD affected kids. Some strategies have been found to be effective in most occasions.

- Note all activity times clearly for the child in visual schedules.
- Use visual choice boards for the child to indicate his/her choice of activity.
- Sometimes, children would have one specific activity that they would prefer to do all the time. In these cases, transition warnings are useful. It may be a timer to let children know that it is time to move on to another activity.
- When doing joint activities like playing, it is important to sometimes accept to undertake activities of other's choices. That makes them respectful of other people's choices.

Sharing

For autistic children, sharing can sometimes be a strange idea and they have difficulties understanding what it means and why it is necessary. The following helps.

- Initially, it is important for the student to understand that he will not lose something by sharing it and that he will be able to participate in using it.

- The concept of when to start and stop comes in handy when explaining the child how to share.
- The caregiver should be aware as to how to repeat the instructions and make the child agree to share.
- When the basics have been learnt, introduce a peer to actually share something.
- Children should be taught to share across activities.

Waiting, taking turns, and playing games

Playing games, waiting and taking turns have to be taught as a part of social behavior and communication skills. Taking turns can be aptly demonstrated with a toy where one is made to share it with others. Waiting can be introduced with a timing device or schedule. Playing games, again, is a social skill where the child should be made to understand that in games, it is okay to lose sometimes and one should not worry about winning or having his/her way all the time.

Chapter 4:
Strategies For Teaching Communication

First of all, autistic children are very different from normal children as far as learning communication skills are concerned. Even among autistic children, there are huge differences as to how each individual learns to communicate. For instance, many autistic children are not comfortable initiating and continuing an effective session of communication.

Around a third of the children affected by ASD fail to develop spoken language skills. Those who manage to pick up spoken language in a meaningful way, have a severely incomplete vocabulary and find it difficult to communicate orally in a functional way. Even when some of them do all the above, they need more time to grasp

what is being said, process it and respond appropriately.
Eye contact is another big issue with these people.
Making normal eye contact and using the gaze properly,
or simply use of eye contact from the body language
perspective is tough for them. These children mostly
avoid eye contact.

Some children may suffer from echolalia, or
repeating words and phrases from previously heard
conversations. Again many autistic children are more
adept at picking up communication skills compared to
others. However, we all should remember that autistic
children have excellent memories and have the
capabilities to acquire excellent vocabularies if trained
properly.

Communicating properly as a social and behavioral
skill is important to everybody and it becomes important
to find out the deficiencies individually. For instance, on
the face of it, it may seem like a student is inattentive or
does not respond to communication from others. The
underlying causes can be many and varied and need to be
understood individually for each child. Maybe the child
has difficulty processing verbal information. It may also
be that the child does not understand the method of
communication being used. In fact, sometimes, it turns
out that the child has heard and understood the
information but is unable to respond appropriately. For
these reasons, a comprehensive assessment by a speech
language pathologist (SLP) is a necessity for each child
and helps find out the area where (like receptive language,
processing, or attention disorders) the child may be

facing difficulties.

A child with ASD can possibly experience the following difficulties:

Following instructions or explanations: This is a specific problem in group settings like classrooms. The child may be busy with non-essential details and may not be 'tuning in' properly.

Understanding popular phrases and expressions: Using expressions like 'she hit the roof' and/or 'get your skates on' or 'you're driving me around the bend' may mislead them because they tend to take things literally. Some expressions, if followed literally can land your precious child in a soup. So, be careful.

Misunderstandings: When somebody says something sarcastic to your child accompanying pleasant body language, other than taking things literally, your child would take the visual cue (the pleasant body language in this case) and might feel happy about it.

Respecting others viewpoints may not come naturally to autistic children. They tend to speak without assessing where the listener is coming from or the listener's knowledge levels. That may be embarrassing sometimes.

Talking around a subject is one of their tendencies and that renders their listeners bored, and at times repetitive and sometimes incoherent.

Recognizing nonverbal communication like body language is an issue with autistic children and the lack of this recognition sometimes lead to a situation, for instance, when they might not realize that a conversation has broken down and they should move on. They cannot alter their conversation to repair the breakdown.

When spoken to as a part of a group, you may face an apparent inattention. They may actually be facing some difficulty in understand what has been said and might be buying time before coming up with a response. It might be worse sometimes and they might not be aware that they are being spoken to. Be prepared and keep checking.

Obsession is sometimes an issue. They sometimes tend to speak about their favorite topic/subject even when that might not be appropriate.

They are unable to successfully ask for help and tend to react to situations inappropriately.

Insensitivity to accepted conditions or conventions of social behavior is displayed by some autistic children while some of them are excellent speakers. Their understanding of humor is also severely limited.

Strategies to help them communicate effectively

- The caregiver should be aware of the student's level of communication and communicate at that level.
- Use simple language that is clearly understood. Use visual support when needed and never use sarcasm.
- Gain the child's attention by talking to the student directly.
- Praise and encourage all attempts by students to communicate.
- Speak slowly and give them the time to understand and comprehend.
- Use familiar words and always make sure that they know how to ask for clarifications when confused.
- Provide the child opportunities to practice their language skills with caregivers, peers and others.
- Guide and prompt the student to respond if needed.
- If the child is a very reluctant communicator, have a home-school notebook where the parents or caregivers at home can communicate with the school staff.
- Persist with any interaction till the desired effect is achieved.

Chapter 5:
Parent Involvment, IEP And An Appropriate Space

Parent involvement

Parents play a very important role in the life and education of ASD affected children. They act like partners for the whole process, providing perspectives, opinions and information about the child, his traits, habits, other feedback, etc.

A collaborative partnership between home and school can be a blessing. Frequent opportunities for discussions and feedback about the child's individual learning needs can indeed make a big positive difference to your child's life. Make sure you are in regular touch with school.

Autistic students have trouble transferring or generalizing knowledge and skills from one situation to another. Of course the child gains most because a collaborative home and school. For him, it means that same skills and concepts are reinforced throughout (at home and school) and leaves little scope for any confusion. A lack of this kind of coordination might bring a lot of confusion to the child's life, often having to learn a separate set of instruction at home and school. It sure makes life a lot better for your child if his parents and teachers share common approach, focus and goals.

These are the main types of valuable information that parents and teachers can share:

- The developmental history of the child.
- Any important health issues.
- Information about the range of professionals and caregivers that have been involved in caring for the child.
- Likes, dislikes, sensory sensitivities, and special interests of the child.
- Knowledge about effective positive reinforces and motivators that work with the child.
- How the child has learnt a particular skill at home.
- Behaviors and strategies that have been successful at home or in other environments.
- Performances as students over brief and long periods

of time and different settings.

- Perspectives on the student's perspectives, and other useful information.

An important to consider the format, information that needs to be shared, and other information that might be needed from the parents by the school on a daily basis. There should be strict guidelines for reporting any significant behavioral changes or events that need mention between home and school. Generally, the classroom teacher is responsible for the content of home school communication. You may consider it a daily diary for the student. Things that should be included in the diary are like:

- Activities in which the student participated.
- Any new skill that was demonstrated to the child.
- The nature of play with classmates.
- Songs and stories of the day.
- New areas of learning.
- Upcoming events, trips or any special interactions/participations.

The Individual Education Plan (IEP)

The Individual Education Plan (or IEP) is a written program or a plan that mentions and describes any special education or service that the student might need.

It is done on the basis of a thorough assessment and understanding of the child's strengths, weakness and/or needs. The information contained in the IEP will guide the caregivers in dealing with the child throughout his education and needs periodic reviews and updates. Almost all students with ASD would need an IEP. It is important that the parents and teachers of the child collaborate and decide on an individualized plan that suits the specific needs of the child. The reviews should take into account the student's performance in assessments during a specified period, like a term, semester or year.

Look at the IEP as a working document that identifies and provide for a child's specific needs as far as educating the child is considered. The IEP also identifies or modifies the alternative learning expectations for the child. Specific knowledge and skills the child is required to be tested for should be mentioned in IEP's. Proper mention and reporting of the child's achievements are necessary. Also, human, technical or other support needed for the child to excel in in general or specific areas should find mention in the IEP.

An effective IEP for a child should be based on his abilities and should gradually increase in terms of complexities involved in completing a task. The program should be based on formal and informal assessments of the child in all or specific areas of learning. And of course, I have already talked of effective periodic reviews. It is one of the first things a parent should be talk of when speaking with the school authorities.

Many children with ASD have issues processing the

information provided to them and are sometimes unable to respond right away and "on demand" to the work or output expected of them. They often need more flexibility as far as the timing and method used to demonstrate the skills and knowledge acquired is concerned. The teachers will need to consider the multiple available alternatives, like extended delivery times and additional activities that may be planned to ensure the most of the required learning experiences are provided to needy students in specific situations. All this should be mentioned in the IEP.

An appropriate space

Arrangement of physical and visual aspects in the learning environment (mostly class) has an important role to play to make life better for them. These children are sometimes sensitive to sensory stimulations and may sometimes overwhelm some children. Distractions should be minimized wherever possible. For instance, the furniture be as noiseless as possible (like a rubber pad at the bottom of the all the furniture's legs).

Students need to be taught where things belong. Organization of their workspace (like keeping pen in a pen stand and files in the file cabinet) can be an important prop in many cases.

Many such adjustments might be necessary at school and home and can only happen when parents collaborate with teachers. Having a plan and sharing it is needed to make the lives of those affected by ASD a lot better.

Chapter 6:
Guideline For Teachers To Teach Students With Autism

Adding to the Personal or Individual Education Plan (IDE)

Designing the personal education plan for the students with autism is really complex because each student has huge contrasts from other student in learning style, correspondence, and social aptitude advancement, what's more, frequently has challenging behaviors.

Programs must be individualized and in light of the unique needs and capacities of every student with autism. Teachers have to judge the capacity of the student with autism to process data and the way of communication before they design an education plan for them. An instruction project could incorporate a mix of instructional exercises from the consistent educational program and in addition exercises in view of objectives and destinations that are exceptional to the individual and set out in nicely an Individual Education Plan.

The IEP is created through cooperation by a group of individuals specifically included with the students with autism, for example, the classroom instructor, grandparents, parents, and custom curriculum instructor. In a few cases, arranging includes others, for example, dialect pathologists, assistants of the teachers, behavior experts, and school clinicians. It is imperative for school staff to be mindful of intercessions being utilized to support their students, so that the school project can be as harmonious as could be allowed with that program or treatment.

The needs of a few students with a mental imbalance and the bolster needed to address those issues once in a while go past the order of the school framework. To be most proficient and have the best results for a student, a communitarian approach among each will be helpful. Some school locale have thought that it was useful to create conventions with neighborhood organizations for how they will cooperate so as to arrangement bolsters for students and their families.

At the point when adding to a student's IEP, it is critical to arrange adjustments to guideline, classroom environment, and classroom administration that address the needs of the student with autism and that will empower him or her to function ideally in the classroom. Correspondence and social abilities are key regions of improvement for students with a mental imbalance and must be tended to in the education plan.

Roles and Responsibilities of Teachers and Family Members

- **Classroom Teachers:** Classroom teachers have the main responsibilities to handle the projects of all students with autism in their classes. At the point when a student with a mental imbalance needs specific programming and direction, class teachers need to work collectively with specialists to guarantee that there is a well-arranged, coordinated methodology.
- **Specialists:** Teachers with special training known as the specialists who must have the working experience with students with autism. They have to understand exceptional needs of the students. Pro instructors have mastery in conduct administration and improvement of social abilities. For a few students with a mental imbalance, the specialist may give direct direction, while in different cases, specialists also give consultative support for classroom teachers who have a student with a mental imbalance in regular class.
- **Family Members:** The family members of students

with autism have information and experience that is significant in adding to a powerful program at school. Family members can answer some questions that are very important to develop a teaching program for a student.

- ✓ What are the weakest points of their child?
- ✓ What makes their child happier and sadder?
- ✓ How they react in different situations and much more.

Steps to Design Individual Teaching Environment

Here are the steps to design IEP

(d) Step One: Educate Yourself

You must have a working comprehension of extreme interconnectedness and what that implies for your specific students. Your knowledge about autism will advance as your association with the family and the student creates and your insight about the issue and abilities in managing its effect on the classroom develops.

(e) Step Two: Reach Out to the Parents

Folks are your first and best wellspring of data about their tyke. Secure a working association with your student's guardians. Building trust with the folks is key. After that, securing commonly concurred modes and examples of correspondence with the family all through the school year is basic.

(f) Step Three: Prepare the Classroom

There are ways you can oblige a percentage of the needs of youngsters with autism in your classroom that will improve their chance to learn without relinquishing your arrangements for the class all in all. Obviously, there are down to earth confinements on the amount you can adjust the physical qualities of your classroom, however even a couple of lodging to bolster a tyke with a mental imbalance may have amazing results.

(g) Step Four: Educate Peers and Promote Social Goals

You must try to advance acknowledgement of the tyke with Autism as a full part and vital piece of the class, regardless of the fact that that understudy just goes to class for a couple of hours a week. As the educator of a tyke with Autism, you must make a social domain that supports positive associations between the kid with a mental imbalance and his or her regularly creating companions for the duration of the day.

(h) Step Five: Collaborate on the Implementation of an Educational Plan

Since your student with Autism has extraordinary needs more than academics, his or her instructive arrangement is characterized by an Individualized Education Program (IEP). The IEP is a diagram for everything that will happen to a tyke in the following school year.

(i) Step Six: Manage Behavioral Challenges

For students with ASD, issue practices may be activated for a mixture of reasons. Such practices may incorporate running about the room, uproarious vocalizations, self-harmful exercises, or other problematic or diverting practices. The key is to be reliable with how you respond to the practices over the long run and to use whatever number positive systems to advance star social practices as could be expected under the circumstances.

Tips for the Teachers to Teach Students with Autism

- Use smart Task Analysis. Need to be very specific. You have to follow a sequential order.

- Continuously keep your language easy to understand. Express what is on your mind in a couple of words as could be expected under the circumstances. Normally, it is significantly more compelling to say "Pens down, close your diary and line up to go outside" than "It looks so decent outside. How about we do our science lesson now. When you've completed your composition, close your books and line up at the entryway. We're going to study plants outside today".

- Show particular social principles/abilities, for example, turn-taking and social separation.

- Give less choices. On the off chance that a tyke is requested that pick a shading, say red, just issue him two to three decisions to pick from. The more decisions, the more confounded an extremely introverted kid will get to be.

- On the off chance that you pose a question or give a direction and are welcomed with a clear gaze, rephrase your sentence. Asking a student with autism what you simply said aides clear up that you've been caught on.

- Abstain from utilizing mockery. On the off chance that an understudy coincidentally thumps every one of your papers on the floor and you say "Awesome!" you will be made truly and this move may be rehashed all the time.

- Abstain from utilizing idioms like "Put your thinking caps on", "Zipper your lips" or "Open your ears" will leave a student with autism totally beguiled and wondering.

Chapter 7:
Parent Guideline To Help A Child With Autism

If you have as of late discovered that your youngster has or may have a mental imbalance range issue, you're most likely pondering and agonizing over what comes next. No guardian is ever arranged to hear that a youngster is something besides glad and solid, and an analysis of Autism can be especially terrifying. You may be uncertain about how to best help your tyke or confounded by clashing treatment guidance. On the other hand you may have been informed that Autism is a hopeless, long lasting condition, abandoning you worried that nothing you do will have any kind of effect.

While beyond any doubt a mental imbalance is not something an individual essentially "develops out of," there are numerous medicines that can help youngsters learn new aptitudes and conquer a wide mixture of formative difficulties. From free taxpayer supported organizations to in-home behavioral treatment and school-based projects, help is accessible to meet your youngster's unique needs. With the right treatment arrangement, and a ton of adoration and backing, your tyke can learn, develop, and flourish.

Guideline for Parents: Things You Have to Do to Support Your Child

As the guardian of a kid with a mental imbalance or related formative defers, the best thing you can do is to begin treatment immediately. Look for help when you think something's incorrectly. Try not to hold up to check whether your kid will look up some other time or exceed the issue. Try not to try and sit tight for an official finding. The prior youngsters with autism range issue get help, the more noteworthy their shot of treatment achievement. Early intercession is the best approach to accelerate your kid's improvement and diminish the manifestations of a mental imbalance.

- **Learn More About Autism Disorder:** The more you think about a mental imbalance range issue, the better prepared you'll be to settle on educated choices for your tyke. Teach yourself about the treatment choices, make inquiries, and take part in all treatment choices.

- **Become a Specialist:** Make sense of what triggers your child's "awful" or problematic practices and what inspires a positive reaction. What does your mentally unbalanced kid find unpleasant? Cooling? Uncomfortable? Agreeable? In the event that you comprehend what influences your tyke, you'll be better at investigating issues and anticipating circumstances that cause challenges.

- **Accept Your Child:** As opposed to concentrating on how your mentally unbalanced kid is unique in relation to other kids and what he or she is "missing," practice acknowledgement. Appreciate your child's exceptional idiosyncrasies, praise little triumphs, and quit contrasting your kid with others. Feeling unequivocally cherished and acknowledged will help your tyke more than whatever else.

- **Try not to Give Up:** It is difficult to foresee the course of a mental imbalance range issue. Try not to make a hasty judgment about what life will be similar to for your kid. Like others, individuals with a mental imbalance have a whole lifetime to develop and build up their capacities.

Tips One for Parents: Create a Safety Zone for Your Child

Gather as much knowledge as you can about Autism and getting included in treatment will go far toward helping your tyke. Also, the accompanying tips will make every day home life simpler for both you and your extremely introverted kid:

Be Steady: Kids with a mental imbalance have some major snags adjusting what they've realized in one setting, (for example, the specialist's office or school) to others, including the home. Case in point, your youngster may utilize gesture based communication at school to convey, however never think to do as such at home. Making consistency in your kid's surroundings is the most ideal approach to strengthen learning. Discover what your tyke's advisors are doing and proceed with their strategies at home. Investigate the likelihood of having treatment occur in more than one spot to urge your tyke to exchange what he or she has gained starting with one environment then onto the next. It's additionally critical to be predictable in the way you associate with your tyke and manage testing practices.

Stick to a Timetable: Youngsters with a mental imbalance have a tendency to do best when they have a profoundly organized calendar or schedule. Once more, this backtracks to the consistency they both need and hunger for. Set up a timetable for your tyke, with consistent times for suppers, treatment, school, and sleep time. Attempt to keep interruptions to this routine to a base. On the off chance that there is an unavoidable timetable change, set up your kid for it ahead of time.

Compensate Good Behavior: Uplifting feedback can run far with youngsters with autism, so attempt to "find them doing something great." Praise them when they act suitably or take in another ability, being certain about what conduct they're being adulated for. Likewise search for different approaches to compensate them for good conduct, for example, issuing them a sticker or giving them a chance to play with a most loved toy.

Make a Home-safety Zone: Cut out a private space in your home where your youngster can unwind, feel secure, and be safe. This will include arranging and defining limits in ways your kid can get it. Visual signs can be useful. You might likewise need to security proof the house, especially if your kid is inclined to fits of rage or other self-harmful practices.

Tips Two for Parents: Learn Nonverbal Way of Communication

Associating with a tyke with Autism can be testing, yet you don't have to talk so as to impart and bond. You impart by the way you take a gander at your tyke, the way you touch him or her, and by the tone of your voice and your non-verbal communication. Your youngster is additionally speaking with you, regardless of the possibility that he or she never talks. You simply need to take in the dialect.

Search for Nonverbal Signs: In the event that you are perceptive and mindful, you can figure out how to get on the nonverbal signals that youngsters with autism utilization to convey. Pay consideration on the sorts of sounds they make, their outward appearances, and the motions they utilize when they're drained, hungry, or need something.

Try to Understand the Needs of Your Child: It is just characteristic to feel upset when you are misconstrued or overlooked, and it is the same for youngsters with autism. At the point when kids with a mental imbalance showcase, it is regularly in light of the fact that you're not getting on their nonverbal signs. Having a fit is their direction conveying their disappointment and standing out enough to be noticed.

Arrange Time for Fun: A youngster adapting to autism is still a child. For both kids with autism and their guardians, there necessities to be more to life than treatment. Plan recess when your youngster is most ready and conscious. Make sense of approaches to have a fabulous time together by contemplating the things that make your youngster grin, chuckle, and leave their shell. Your youngster is liable to appreciate these exercises most in the event that they don't appear to be remedial or instructive. There are gigantic advantages that outcome from your delight in your kid's organization and from your tyke's satisfaction in investing unpressurized energy with you. Have a crucial impact of learning and shouldn't feel like work.

Pay Attention on the Sensitiveness of Your Child: Numerous youngsters with a mental imbalance are touchy to light, solid, touch, taste, and smell. Other kids with a mental imbalance are "under-touchy" to tangible boosts. Make sense of what sights, sounds, scents, developments, and material sensations trigger your child's "terrible" or troublesome practices and what inspires a positive reaction. What does your extremely introverted tyke find distressing? Cooling? Uncomfortable? Pleasant? On the off chance that you comprehend what influences your kid, you'll be better at investigating issues, anticipating circumstances that cause challenges, and making effective encounters.

Tips Three for Parents: Create a Personal Treatment Plan for Your Child

With such a large number of diverse a mental imbalance medicines accessible, and it can be hard to make sense of which approach is ideal for your youngster. Making things more confused, you may hear diverse or notwithstanding clashing suggestions from folks and specialists. At the point when assembling an autism treatment arrangement for your youngster, remember that there is no single treatment that will work for everybody. Every individual on a mental imbalance range is novel, with distinctive qualities and shortcomings. Your youngster's treatment ought to be customized by or her individual needs. You know your tyke best, so its dependent upon you to verify those needs are being met.

Remember that regardless of what a mental imbalance treatment arrangement is picked, your inclusion is essential to achievement. You can help your tyke get the most out of treatment by meeting expectations as one with the autism treatment group and finishing the treatment at home.

Concerning a mental imbalance treatment, there are a confounding mixture of treatments and methodologies. Some a mental imbalance treatments concentrate on lessening tricky practices and building correspondence and social abilities, while others manage tactile mix issues, engine aptitudes, intense subject matters, and nourishment sensitivities.

With such a large number of decisions, it is amazingly critical to do your examination, converse with a mental imbalance treatment specialists, and make inquiries. At the same time, remember that you don't need to pick only one sort of treatment. The objective of autism treatment ought to be to treat the majority of your kid's side effects and needs. This frequently obliges a joined treatment approach that exploits a wide range of sorts of treatment.

Regular autism medicines incorporate conduct treatment, discourse dialect treatment, play-based treatment, active recuperation, word related treatment, and nutritious treatment.

Tips Four for Parents: Find Support and Help for Your Child

Caring for Autistic can request a ton of vitality and time. There may be days when you feel overpowered, focused on, or demoralized. Child rearing isn't ever simple, and bringing up a youngster with exceptional needs is significantly additionally difficult. So as to be the best parent you can be, it is key that you deal with yourself. Try not to attempt to do everything all alone. You don't need to! There are numerous spots that groups of extremely introverted children can swing to for guidance, some assistance, support and advocacy:

Autism Care Groups: Joining a mental imbalance care group is an extraordinary approach to meet different families managing the same difficulties you are. Folks can impart data, get counsel, and incline toward one another for enthusiastic backing. Simply being around others in almost the same situation and imparting their experience can go far toward diminishing the seclusion numerous folks feel in the wake of getting a tyke's a mental imbalance determination.

Break Care: Every guardian needs a break every so often. Also, for folks adapting to the included anxiety of a mental imbalance, this is particularly genuine. In rest consideration, another guardian assumes control briefly, showing you an a bit of mercy for a couple of hours, days, or even weeks. To discover break care alternatives in your general vicinity.

Individual, Conjugal, or Family Guiding: If anxiety, tension, or sorrow is getting to you, you may need to see your very own specialist. Treatment is a sheltered spot where you can speak sincerely about all that you're feeling—the great, the terrible, and the appalling. Marriage or family treatment can likewise bail you work out issues that the difficulties of existence with a mentally unbalanced tyke are creating in your spousal relationship.

Conclusion

In conclusion, I would like to talk about Applied Behavior Analysis (ABA), which you can think of as an instructional approach to effectively teach these people any skill. ABA uses methods of instruction based on scientific principles of learning and behavior.

First the behavior to be changed is clearly defined. And then, any possible reinforcements and antecedents encouraging this behavior are changed with repeated and focused methods of instructions. If needed, any new skills that might help them change the identified behavior can also be taught.

Once again, the individual is the key here. ABA can and should be used in conjunction with an IEP. The IEP should clearly state the behaviors to be modified or the ones that are being worked upon right now. The ultimate goal of ABA should be to help the student generalize any skill he has learnt and use it according to varying situations and places.

In fact, for those genuinely interested in being a great caregiver or parent, knowing the basics of ABA is absolutely necessary for

- Increasing positive behaviors and decreasing negative ones.
- Teaching new skills.
- Maintain the positive ones already learnt.

- Narrow down and restrict the conditions under which an interfering behavior occurs and
- Helping the student generalize and understand how new skills/behaviors can be generalized and used across situations.

If you are serious about parenting, teaching or caring for a child affected with ASD, ABA is something you must know.

Thank you for reading this book! I hope it was able to help you. Finally, if you enjoyed this book, then I'd like to ask you for a favor, would you be kind enough to leave a positive review for it on Amazon? It'd be greatly appreciated!

I want to share this book and help as many people as I can, and more reviews will help me accomplish that!

I wish you the best of luck.

Suzanne Jensen

ALL RIGHTS RESERVED. No part of this publication may be reproduced or transmitted in any form whatsoever, electronic, or mechanical, including photocopying, recording, or by any informational storage or retrieval system without express written, dated and signed permission from the author.

DISCLAIMER AND/OR LEGAL NOTICES:

Every effort has been made to accurately represent this book and it's potential. Results vary with every individual, and your results may or may not be different from those depicted. No promises, guarantees or warranties, whether stated or implied, have been made that you will produce any specific result from this book. Your efforts are individual and unique, and may vary from those shown. Your success depends on your efforts, background and motivation.

The material in this publication is provided for educational and informational purposes only and is not intended as medical advice. The information contained in this book should not be used to diagnose or treat any illness, metabolic disorder, disease or health problem. Always consult your physician or health care provider before beginning any nutrition or exercise program. Use of the programs, advice, and information contained in this book is at the sole choice and risk of the reader.

Manufactured by Amazon.ca
Bolton, ON